THE SLEEP GAME

how to win a night's rest

FOLLOWING A PERSONAL tragedy in 1945, the author found it imperative to discover a reliable way of inducing sleep. Her profession of journalist was at risk; indeed, she feared for her sanity.

SOME SIMPLE RULES found in a digest helped Vida Heard attain a certain degree of relaxation. As time went by she began adapting them to her own requirements and eventually formulated the 'Repose Recipe' that forms the nuculeus of her supremely helpful method.

DEMONSTRATIONS TO UNIVERSITY students convinced Vida Heard that people of all age groups could benefit from her teaching. So she wrote this book, which was first published in her home country of South Africa. Letters of appreciation poured in from men and women who found the 'Repose Recipe' provided a happy release from the torture of insomnia.

READERS ARE ASKED to note that to gain maximum benefit from this book they should read it through *three* times before commencing their nightly practice of the 'Repose Recipe'.

THE SLEEP GAME

how to win a night's rest

THE
SLEEP GAME
how to win a night's rest

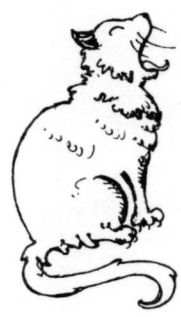

by VIDA HEARD

Decoration: BRENDA LIGHTON

THORSONS PUBLISHERS LIMITED
37/38 Margaret Street, London W.1

Originally published by Happy Life Books,
Cape Town, Republic of South Africa 1969

First English Edition March 1972

ISBN 0 7225 0191 9

Typeset by Specialised Offset Services, Liverpool.
and printed by Weatherby Woolnough Ltd.,
Sanders Road, Wellingborough, Northampton.

Contents

Foreword

It's smartly smug to debunk self-cures. For long auto-suggestion has been OUT, and IN have been the instant cure-alls, the pills, in vicarious variety.

Yet the pendulum shows signs of a swing back. The IN methods have already had too long an innings and modern psychology preaches it's not too difficult to replace one habit (bad) by another habit (good). For this reason the writer passes on to others the simple natural relaxation methods she evolved to defeat insomnia when wrestling with a tragic mystery (never solved) in her own life.

Her compulsion to write this book? A year spent recently in Washington, D.C., in an affluent community whose 'pills-bills' were fantastic and reliance on artificial aids pathetic — even for their domestic pets.

Her market research? Just people: a lifetime editing various women's magazines in Southern Africa, dealing with hundreds of human problems.

And this is the result: A light-hearted book which, while in parts is amusing, nevertheless claims to solve a serious personal problem — the fear of sleeplessness.

For success the reader should not skip a word and study to saturation point the vital chapter *Recipe for Repose*.

VIDA HEARD

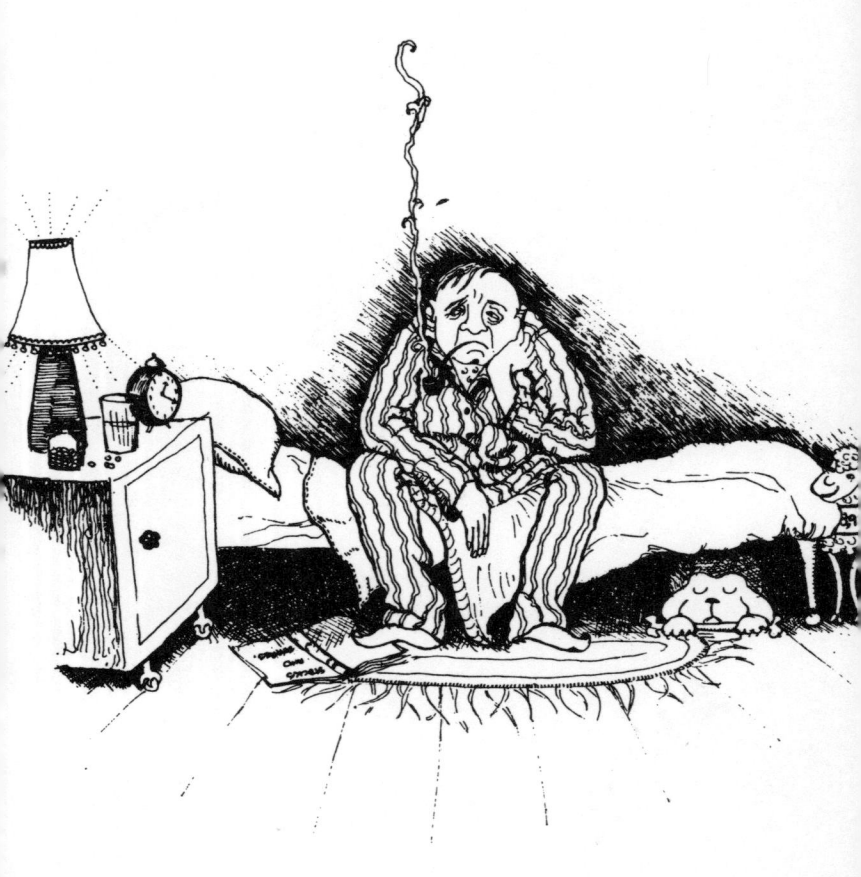

If you are happy in your sleepless state, don't read on.

1

What is Your Attitude to Sleep?

If you are happy in your sleepless state, don't read on. If you could not bear to be able to say, 'I slept well last night', when others around you moan they had a 'terrible night', this book is not for you. Insomnia may have become a status claim you hate to destroy, or you may have hypnotized yourself into actually believing you are an insomniac. But if you really must — drastically *must* sleep — or else? Or if you have decided a pill is only a crutch and not the answer; if you are convinced that learning to sleep naturally will make you a better adjusted person, more healthy, more successful, longer lived, and nicer to live with, then turn these pages for future happiness.

There are many people who are convinced they don't sleep, when actually they do, and for longer than they think they do. Tests with students in the U.S.A. revealed that when awakened after one hour most were unable to guess how long they had slept. Others, conscious of tossing and turning and waking at intervals, are harassed by the thought that they are light sleepers and should be heavier sleepers. The message of this book will help them too, persuading them that heavy sleeping is not so desirable as it may seem; persuading them that once they have the right attitude, every minute of wakefulness and sleepfulness is cherished, releasing them forever from the fears of not sleeping as much as they feel they ought to do.

To the child — father of the man — who sleeps 'like a log' the contents of this book may read like nonsense. Of course, this was not written for anyone who sleeps regularly, normally and happily. It was written by request of those who have asked me how I learnt to sleep to overcome mulling over every night a tragic mystery in my own family life. And how little did I realise over twenty years ago, when I first started out on this sleep method, that it would actually work in my case. Because my need was desperate enough I had to find a way out. And I did, but half heartedly at first, without any inkling that I was on the threshold of something that would change my whole life. My source was a few pages, a condensation of a book in *The Readers Digest* (I've no idea of the title). To stave off a further nervous breakdown and continue working (for the sake of myself and my children) I practised the few basic rules given on how to sleep without pills. From this, through the years, I built success not only for my own sleeping but that of many others in all age groups — as recounted in relevant chapters.

The first thing the reader will notice is that this book is cluttered with repetitions and trivialities; repetition of the method as we go along and repetition of the telling of the method and its application. It took me a long time to realise that this repetition is the secret of the success of the application for sleep education, as also of the telling. I am sure there are many people armed with quite as good relaxation systems who could apply them equally successfully as I did, but find they do not work out because of some missing links, little things so trivial that one hesitates to commit them to paper. These small details I have found can be of vital importance in the sleep study . . . and for this reason they are all here — in case some reader has tried before and given up in despair because his relaxation system didn't work. These details, tiny links in the chain, I've found cannot be extracted, without the chain itself breaking apart.

In these pages you will not find any reference to advertised sleep inducers, tick-tocking instruments, mattresses, pillows, drugs or special beds. This method does not rely on anything but your own regular application to a relaxation drill — the *Repose Recipe*, chapter 6. If you sleep on a feather bed or on hard ground, the same applies. I do admit that sleeping in the same bed with anyone else might fail you in your first attempts; the lesson repeated every night does need concentration on the lesson itself and nothing less. It is only when the sleep lesson is learnt that you can ignore or tend others, or do as you wish by cutting up or prolonging your sleep, as you yourself decide and desire.

Yes, this all sounds *Svengali* and rather absurd to those who sleep well and naturally; it may also seem trite to some medical men and psychologists; 'all this is well known' they say. My answer is, then why is it that so many people, including themselves, are victims of sleeplessness? Why is it that medical men give out so many pills to so many patients? There is an answer, of course, but it is not the answer given in this 'natural' sleep course.

The aim of this book is to describe a method to promote natural sleep. Natural sleep is not a deep sleep — unless one is dog tired. Yet, talking of dogs, they can sleep almost anytime they want to — when bored, depressed, too full or too hungry; see how they curl round and round until they are comfortable, shut off excess oxygen with their paws, and then snooze off. A very exhausted dog twitches and even barks in his sleep; but dog-tired or not, he (and most other animals) never sleep so soundly that they are unaware when danger threatens. Our dachshund was awakened by the smell of smoke when a fire broke out in the next garden and 'barked her head off', thereby enabling us to call the fire brigade in time to save the houses around; the fantastic thing is that she slept with a blanket over her head. Dogs and other creatures, while appearing to sleep soundly, wake quickly to give warning of any strange noise, then when they are satisfied there is no danger, they settle down to slumber again. It is this *natural* sleep, that can be interrupted and yet resumed at will, that we seek; as in a parent's case to awake to a child's cry, tend the child and relax to sleep again.

With drugs and other artificial ways of promoting sleep one is not usually as able to minister to a sick person or waken easily to be aware of danger. No one in his right senses, enjoying natural sleep, for example, would fall asleep and leave a burning cigarette on the bed. But this is a far too common occurrence when drugs have been taken.

Here is a way to capture the simple sleep of a child, the revitalizing 'animal sleep' where one dozes off while guarding the young; the life-prolonging, natural sleep that every bread-winner needs — forgetting office and business worries, he wakes in the morning refreshed and able to tackle them and, as sometimes happens, with a solution to the problem born of sleep! Many famous men bearing the weight of the world on their shoulders have been able to turn 'sleep on and off' as required, Napoleon, Edison and Churchill among them; and because of their ability to control sleep, they seemed to require less than other men. Lady Baden Powell in her 81st year said, 'I've no aches and pains and can sleep well anywhere'. That's our ideal at any age.

2

Excuses…Why I Can't Sleep

The Human Comedy

From inquiry among my friends these seem to be some of the more usual excuses, with my answers:

I've too active a brain.

Good for you; it's a better brain than an inactive one. It will be better still when you learn to relax it by practising the *Repose Recipe*, chapter 6.

I have so many worries at the office. Everything depends on me. If I cave in, the family will too.

Learn to sleep naturally, after making a list of your assets and your worries (liabilities). I remember thinking, 'how can I educate my children?' — one of my chief worries — but they educated themselves even to Honours degrees (I never thought of that!) Whatever the worries, we are able to face them and make a plan to eliminate them when we enjoy healthy sleep to restore our vitality, optimism and faith.

My bladder is weak and I have to get up several times each night.

Read carefully to the last page and you will see how this problem makes no difference.

I've a conscience and each night it blackmails me.

You are in excellent company; it's a millionaire's malady. 'The sleep of a labouring man is sweet, whether he eat little or much; but the abundance of the rich will not suffer him to sleep', according to Ecclesiastes, Chapter 5, verse 12. This teach-yourself-to-sleep method applies to the rich man as well as those worrying how they can get rich.

I'm getting on — will be 92 next birthday. I dread going to bed.

Before you read this book further turn to the chapter on Old Age. It may help.

My indigestion keeps me awake. I have always suffered severe flatulence and although doctors tell me not to worry I'm in such discomfort I find it hard to sleep.

You, like the chronic cramp sufferers, come under medical supervision; but those considered normally healthy may be helped by the Chapter *Comfort*, page 46.

My husband snores.

Yes, you may need separate rooms, but unless you practise the sleep formula it will still be a sleepless problem for you, even in your own room. (See Chapter 7. *Some Special Cases.*)

I'm dieting and get terribly hungry in the night . . . this keeps me awake.

The compulsive eater and dieter both have a real problem here, yet it is not unsolvable. (See particularly *Comfort* Chapter and *Special Cases* and read to the end.)

I'm particularly highly strung, and hear every noise in the night.

Good for you if you have to be on guard (or responsible for a sick person); as I was once responsible for keeping up the fire to keep the elephants away from our tiny tent in one of the Game reserves. I admit it is good to be highly strung, to be on tiptoe and on your guard; but the joy of acquiring the mastery of sleep is that you can doze between throwing wood on a camp fire, looking after a sick child, or like Winston Churchill did — fight a war and govern a nation succoured by the ability to catnap.

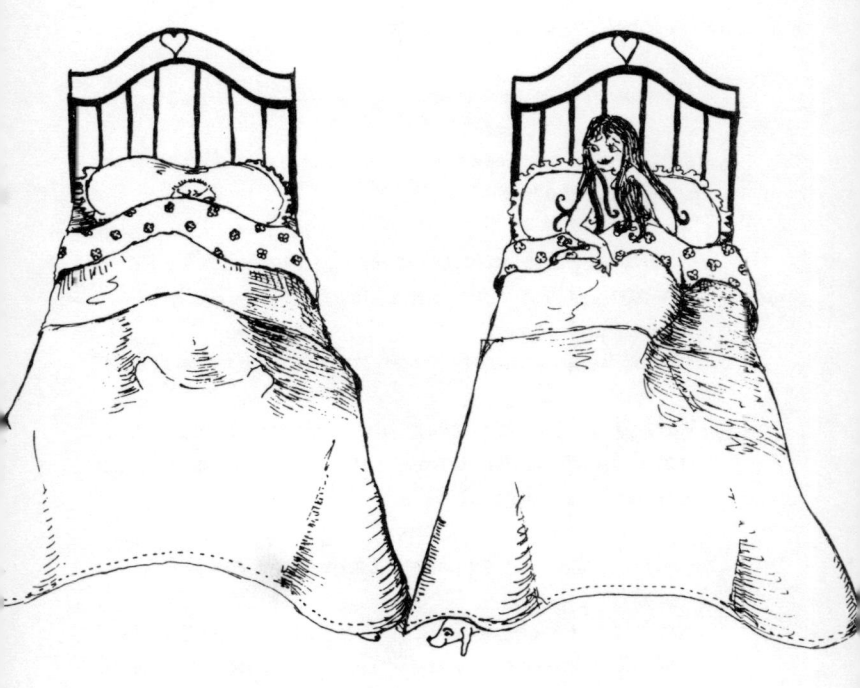

Must we have separate beds?

My husband is not what he should be; he falls asleep satisfied while I toss and turn, completely frustrated and unhappy.

Even with the aid of a marriage guidance counsellor, you are still advised to learn to sleep.

My wife ditto (less often reported).

The answer is as above.

I have been an insomniac from childhood; how can I change the pattern?

It is never too late to learn, anyway this side of Seventy. (Over that, see Chapter *Old Age*).

Must we have separate beds to practise relaxation?

Yes, but less divorces have resulted from separate beds than when one partner is an insomniac or taker of pills.

I've suffered so much, more than most people.

'Still last to come where thou are wanted most', said Wordsworth who wrote a whole sonnet to Sleep. That's why you need to learn to sleep — more than most people.

I have an impossible family; baby two months, child of eighteen months, older children of three, six and nine and my husband is on nightwork. I'm always tired but never seem to have a chance of sleeping properly anytime.

You are actually better off than most mothers because you at least have the night to yourself. Practise the *Repose Recipe* every night and save yourself increased suffering in later years.

We live next to a busy highway, motor cycles scream all night . . . Jets thunder overhead . . . we have terribly noisy people in the flat above and/or below . . . etc.

The same reply to all these: Realise it is resentment, anger that is keeping you awake. Buy comfortable ear plugs and/or ear muffs and follow the formula given here, including all the background stuff. The resentment of your noisy neighbours will diminish and the awful noises recede to become just a hum.

There's nothing really wrong with me (I'm a commercial traveller) but after a long drive I can't get to sleep; I'm driving the car right through the night, pulling up at stop signs, dodging weavers, and missing an abyss by a hairbreadth.

You are just one of the many that the pressure of modern living is getting down; but just think of the train driver or air pilot; if he finds himself driving in imagination all night the sign is that he is becoming a nervous wreck. This system of natural sleep is a natural salvation for you — and for them.

I cannot sleep in a strange bed. Away from home I feel restless at night — however excellent the hotel mattress may be.

It is not the bed so much as your attitude to being away from home, fear or irritation when in a new environment, or maybe excitement resulting from over-stimulating conditions during the day or evening; alcohol or food in excess. When you have mastered the *Repose Recipe* such discomforts will be overcome. Refer to the Chapter on *Comfort*.

My teenage children go out at night and I cannot sleep, thinking of what might happen to them. I lie awake until I hear them safely in the house.

Parents who suffer from this age-old malady might well consider if their lying awake will safeguard the offspring who, incidentally, may be of any age from fourteen on, even twenty and more than eligible to vote! This special problem is not easily solved but, for the sake of the teenager and parent, it must be tackled. One psychologist suggests: Firstly, the parent should impress the child with his interest in his activities and his love for him, *whatever* should happen. Secondly, trust the child to tell at breakfast time what time he came in and encourage him to recount his adventures, even party pranks. (This sometimes works but not always.) Thirdly, see that the child has an identification disc on wrist or neck (these are fashionable anyway) or some card with name and address and telephone number, and explain that the phone is next to your bed if he needs you at any time. No more can you do — except to practise your *Repose Recipe* and go to sleep naturally with a view to a happy future for the whole family, including yourself. Over-anxious parents become impossible parents-in-law!

I've not slept well since I was put on night shifts; although I wear ear-plugs and a night mask to shield the light.

Here again the complainant is suffering from anxiety — a self-hypnosis that he cannot sleep. Yet actually the daylight noises can be less irksome than those night ones when the stillness is suddenly pierced by aircraft overhead or siren of ambulance or fire engine. It is interesting to note that people at the poles who have months of daylight do apparently sleep adequately. For his own happiness and that of the family he should not try to 'hush' all those around him. They must lead normal lives, and his can also be a normal life. He is advised to read this book in every detail, taking particular cognisance of the Chapter on *Comfort*. Continue to wear the

ear-plugs and night mask at least to begin with;
soon you will find you can discard them and
sleep anytime anywhere, as *you* will.

I suffer from what the doctor says is arthritis;
while at work in a busy departmental store during
the day I'm hardly aware of discomfort, but at
night when I go to bed the pain in my joints keeps
me awake.

Far worse cases than yours have benefited by
relaxation exercises. I recently met a woman
who was so crippled with arthritis that she used
sticks; yet she travels throughout the world (by
air, of course). She was one of those who
encouraged me to write this book, for she told
me she had practised a similar relaxation
formula for years and that's why she was free to
visit her friends in other countries, and not be
chained to her apartment — with all the loneli-
ness that would entail. She was under medical
care, of course, and at times had to take the
necessary sedatives prescribed when the pain
became intense. 'Yet I send myself to sleep most
nights by practising relaxation,' she said, 'the
pain is minimized when I am completely relaxed
and concentrating on the relaxation procedure
limb by limb — call it self-hypnotism or what
you will, your *Repose Recipe* does work, even
with such cases as mine.'

I go off to sleep almost immediately my head

touches the pillow, but waken in three or four hours and sometimes do not go off again until almost the time for getting up and going to office. I'm always tired.

This common complaint can arise from various causes. Firstly, the few initial hours of sleep followed by hours of wakefulness has become a habit. To break the habit, as your psychiatrist will tell you, you must replace it with another habit. How? Study the Chapter on *Comfort*.

When you awake how do you feel physically? Are you hungry, or have you a heavy head or stomach resulting from too much food or drink? Or are you merely uncomfortable in your nightwear, curlers or bedding? Get rid of the cause (even if it means being sick!), then practise the *Repose Recipe*. In time you'll break the old habit and find that you will sleep longer — and have banished for ever the *fear* you'll wake up in the night.

Every night when I go to bed I pine for the fellowship and comfort of another human being. I long so much that I lie awake.

According to Nature's plan, the answer is to get married if you can but hoping that you do, remember that even before, as well as forever after marriage, the sleep formula should be yours to fall back on. This book should help you as much as all the others. Indeed, once you have defeated the ogre of insomnia you become a much better adjusted person, more on the ball and lively, more attractive — more *likely* to find a mate.

My husband (or wife) snatches the bed clothes; I lie awake because I'm cold. He likes his feet tucked in and I like mine loose to wiggle my toes. She likes the windows open and I prefer them closed.

All these marital problems cannot be solved by love alone — separate beds or even rooms may be indicated. Read on and don't miss the Chapter *Comfort*.

Other excuses . . . imaginary but probable

(Continuing our Human Comedy)

I lie awake and worry because:
I'm ugly (or old) I feel everyone hates me . . .

I'm rather good looking (she means stunning) and everyone (male gender) worries me to death.

I married my husband for love but now realise he wants me to cook, too.

I'm in an office and counted so low they will not

even let me make the tea and yet I know I could tell the director how to brew better profits.

I'm so lonesome I lie awake all night thinking of how lonesome I am.

My wife, in her latter years, has become even more fond of dogs; at night I have to go to bed with three Basset hounds on my feet. Every time one scratches a flea I itch; then my wife wakes up and asks why I'm so fidgety?

All this sounds like amusing nonsense. Yet, every one of these cases is authentic and might be summed up in the one word FRUSTRATION.

The answer to frustration is simply the same as all the rest, follow the formula; but I insist that the man with three dogs and a wife in his bed must demand his own bed so that he can be free to practise the *Repose Recipe* — otherwise he'll never learn how to sleep naturally!

3

When do You Want to Sleep?

The Comfortable Half State

You want to sleep, instead of suffering some of those mental aches and pains listed in the previous chapter, *Excuses?* But there are the *occasions* and events contained in mere everyday living, when knowing how to run sleep on and off like a water tap, becomes a dream come true. For example, think of long distance travel, by bus, train or plane. Nowadays I enjoy any form of travelling because I doze off when I want to, and have no fear of air travel because I sleep whenever I feel afraid.

On a recent air trip to Europe I was sandwiched between a Japanese business man and a Greek woman and we had such an animated conversation via French that in two hours we were utterly exhausted. The Japanese (next the window) said politely, 'Excuse, now I sleep'. I noticed that he did, as I have learnt to do: just relaxed and went off to sleep; his head tilted back slightly, his jaw dropped, his hands relaxed. (The routine once learnt as described in our key chapter need only be followed in imagination; you cannot lie down, for example, when seated in a plane or bus, but *having learnt* the routine you can adapt to any position that is reasonably comfortable.)

I slept until we were wakened by the air hostess and refreshed with hot towels at midnight to land at Entebbe. But I felt sorry for my Greek woman who had been very quietly sick and tended by the stewardess and who was, apparently very frightened. When we got back into the plane, I said to her — 'try sleep'. She did try, but had no idea of the way to relax, and our language difficulty forbade me describing my *Repose Recipe* in detail. I had not the temerity to ask our Japanese companion to describe his! (No wonder his kind is winning world markets!)

When you know how to sleep you feel desperately sorry for those who cannot draw on this wonderful natural restorative for living a full life. Once you have mastered the sleep routine, it comes to your aid right through life, and everywhere, under all kinds of uncomfortable conditions. Now, think of hospitals, ugh. I'm a particularly bad subject. The bed is so 'overmade' that I cannot kick out the sheets. I feel hamstrung, miserable and bound like a captive in a cage, best summed up by the predicament of men in the film *Planet of the Apes*. I pay honest tribute to surgeons the only three times in my life I have ever been in hospital, but I'm an individual and I have mastered one thing, the importance and joy of natural sleep. Back to the hospital.

The night before a major operation, I undressed and fell asleep between cool sheets — after kicking off the binding blankets round my feet. The anaesthetist, accompanied by the sister in charge, came round that night. The sister hastily summoned a nurse to make me 'respectable' (tuck in my feet) while he, the anaesthetist, checked me according to routine and handed out, with a benevolent smile, the tranquillizer pill. When I thanked him but said I did not want it — 'I can sleep without a pill', he looked at me a trifle hard, blinked behind his glasses then said in a rather disparaging tone, 'Oh you are one of those yogi types'; and left. I felt I was some peculiar 'down-under' being; one who refused his pill was evidently not his class of patient; someone who had no need of his services. (And yet how gratefully one submits to the services of the anaesthetist on the day of the operation!) But somehow I'd rather he had smiled, even if he did not wish to congratulate me for saving the hospital the cost of the tranquillizer pill. Probably I paid for it anyway.

But that Yoga? Maybe I've missed something in not going to Yoga classes. Maybe not, because many of my Yogi friends cannot sleep — although at least one answers phone calls standing on her head. I saw an advertisement recently claiming to teach Yoga and weight-reducing in the right spots. In defence of this true art which I have not practised, it is a science and should not be associated with reducing in any spots. But as it happens, when you learn to sleep simply this natural way, Yoga is unnecessary — although and perhaps not paradoxically, a true Yogi knows how to sleep.

Apart from hospitals and the subject of Yoga, every reader can think of scores of times when he or she longed to drowse off; when the narrator at the Club bores, when the children are tiresome, when you are baby-sitting (see Chapter *Children*). But when you can turn sleep on and off like a water tap, you have attained an accomplishment that will be with you the rest of your life, for in better or in worse, you have reached indeed a state more perfect than Nirvana. Who wants nothingness all the time?

To me the real joy of living is to live fully on tiptoe every minute of the day, and to drift off into peaceful slumber at night or during the day into a half-sleep when I want to. For example, on the bus when shielded by your dark glasses (if not by nodding head) you can be relaxed during a boring conversation about whether the weather will, etcetera; and merely smile, with punctuations, 'how nice', 'shame', 'oh, not so nice, sorry' . . . This is the delightful half-sleep state — that you can assume any time, anywhere, when you feel the need to escape boring or unpleasant experiences.

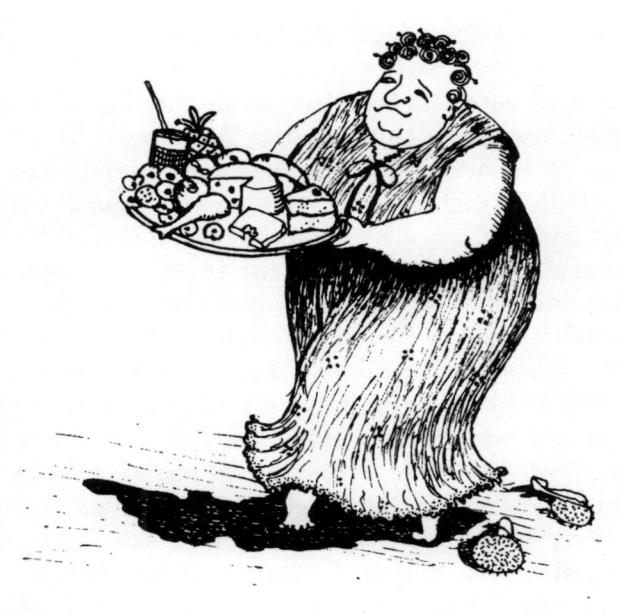

Night-eaters are often overweight people who are compelled to eat because they lie awake thinking about food.

4

Sleep...How Much and What Kind?

Hypnosis and Pill Addiction

It is an accepted fact that people the world over employ about one-third of their lives asleep. While some adults need ten hours (and need not be fools for all that) eight hours is the accepted norm for most and less, say six or seven hours, is what a lot of people get whether they wish it or not. People differ widely as to their sleep requirements, which depend largely on the actual quality of their sleep. And while there are fakirs and monks who can live on four hours of sleep, no culture has been found of people who remain awake all the time; every man, bird and beast sleeps part of his life-span in some way or other. Although some creatures, such as many quadrupeds as well as birds, sleep erect, man, who must support his long spine on only two legs, really needs to lie flat, at least a portion of every twenty-four hours. Sleep is a simple necessity, a law of nature for all.

Primitive man fell asleep readily, as do most men and women who work physically hard during the day. It is the more highly civilized and nervous *homo sapiens* who sleeps less easily and because he knows it is imperative for his health that he sleeps adequately, he has developed an unholy fear of *not* being able to sleep. This has encouraged the night-club habit, the desire to be awake all night, the pushing of bed-time away from him as a waste of time.

This cultivated fear that they will not be able to sleep is passed on by parents to their unfortunate children. Every day you hear mothers say, 'My children musn't sleep during the day or they will not sleep at night.' You, too, must know many people who keep themselves, and their children, awake during the day in aid of a good sleep at night. But all these strivings to 'wear out' the body and tire the brain may actually over-tire the body and brain, making sleep even more hard to come by when one retires to bed at night. 'Relax during the day and you'll sleep better at night', is something many over-tense parents have still to learn . . . and pass on to their children.

Far more effective than trying to tire oneself out is to learn the joy of relaxation during the day, turning sleep on and off; taking a nap in the afternoon if one wishes to, without fear of its subtracting from the full eight hours sleep at night.

The *Repose Recipe* defeats fear; fear of staying awake, which is half the trouble in the case of insomniacs and those who resort to pills. Knowledge is the antidote to fear: cast out fear and learn to sleep at no cost but the learning. Now many people talk about this learning; they have read this book and that, they attend Yoga classes, may quote far better than I have done on the subject of how to relax; and yet if you happen to stay with them in their homes you will find them walking about at night, going to the fridge for food, pulling their hair and the bathroom chain, tossing and turning and moaning in misery — because sleep eludes them. Instead of all these goings-on they might as well practise regularly the relaxation that they *know* — like the five-finger exercises of the beginner at the piano — persevering every night until the body obeys the lesson; the lesson apparently only civilized man must seek.

Deep sleep is often unnatural sleep, especially when the result of sedatives or drugs. Deep sleep is not even the best kind of sleep. According to recent research on dreams it is suggested that dreams are a necessary part of happy, natural sleep and those people who are put into heavy sleep by long-term courses of barbiturates may suffer mentally because they are deprived of their dreaming time! There are those exceptions, of course, where a sedative may be used temporarily by a doctor, as a crutch to induce a sleep habit. But here we are not concerned with these exceptions, only with the normal, reasonably healthy person who wants to establish a natural sleep pattern and thereby be able to cope with all life's emergencies in between.

When you have conquered the fear of not sleeping you will know the joy of relaxation whereby you can operate drowsily. Believe it or not, 'drowsily does it'. There is a way of walking the floor at night with cramp, tending a sick person, even putting the cat out and returning to bed — all in a drowse — resuming sleep forthwith. To fully understand this consider the power of hypnosis.

Hypnotism

The efficient hypnotist can send the most wide-awake characters to sleep at any time and in almost any position, as is frequently demonstrated on the stage.

I'll never forget an evening spent with a friend of mine who was a cinema manager in Natal. A 'showman' hypnotist had been engaged to do his act after the interval, just before the main picture. When the hypnotist invited members from the audience to come up on the stage, my friend, the manager, became slightly alarmed — as up rushed some of his difficult patrons, the teenage types he always kept an eye on to subdue caterwauling and discourage damage to seats. But, to our amazement, in a few minutes the hypnotist had selected six of these rough-house boys and, in a few minutes more, had them all peacefully asleep with the most angelic expressions on their faces. He then got them to perform silly acts, such as removing their socks, sucking a baby's dummy, and so on. My friend said, 'Here's the answer. He must come here again.'

Anyone who has watched a hypnotist do his act will agree the power he has over his subject is almost unbelievable; but, as was explained to me by a medically approved hypnotist, only some people prove suitable subjects; there is no such thing as a hypnotic gaze; neither is it true that the hypnotist has extraordinary will power; he merely knows from experience that his selected subject will obey his commands.

Every hypnotist, apparently, uses more or less the same method to put his subject to sleep. First, he asks him to gaze at a moving object or at a light, or into his eyes — to create a slight strain on the eyes. When he notices that his subject wants to close his eyes he says clearly and convincingly such words as . . . 'your eyes are growing tired, they are getting heavier, heavier, your arms are growing heavier, heavier . . .' (following similar commands in our *Repose Recipe*). 'Now you are growing very tired and going into a deep, sound sleep. Breathe slowly, breathe deeply; you are going deeper and deeper asleep with every breath you take. Nothing will waken you until I waken you.' Or words to that effect. And, for instance, when the hypnotist says 'your right arm is as rigid as steel and you cannot move it', the subject will be unable to move his arm. (Whereas when we practise our *Repose Recipe* for relaxation, while the limbs do become heavy we still *retain our will power* to move them to answer the 'phone, the cry of a child, or anything we feel we are obliged to do — drowsily yet intelligently!)

The readers who have seen the showmen hypnotists in action will realise the tremendous power of suggestion. Yet, as professional hypnotists explained to me: it is not the hypnotist who makes the subject's arm rigid or who puts him to sleep, it is the subject who does it himself by *believing* what the hypnotist tells him. In the same way we often hypnotise ourselves that we cannot sleep naturally according to one of those excuses in the second chapter — and often alas, to our own disadvantage throughout life.

The *Oxford Dictionary* defines hypnotism (shortened from the original *neuro-hypnotism* and derived from the Greek word meaning 'to sleep') as a 'process of hypnotising or artificially producing a state in which the subject appears to be in a deep sleep, without any power of changing his mental or physical condition, except under the influence of some external influence or suggestion.'

Particularly enlightening are the words 'external influence'. The professional hypnotist, when required to help extreme cases, can influence the sub-conscious minds of his patients to a wonderful and often very beneficial degree. But we are concerned only with the average man, woman or child who is not ill, mentally or physically, who can use the amazing powers of hypnotic suggestion for him- or herself. Further, while a subject can be made to do or think all kinds of things outside his own will under hypnosis, you who practise and master the natural way to sleep will have the added satisfaction that all is of your volition. *Why hand over to others what you can do yourself?*

Anyone of normal intelligence and average health can benefit by his own positive thinking, safely within his own religious beliefs and without offending anyone, especially if his partner (who may be a good sleeper) reads this book too, in encouragement. Yet here let it be stressed that only the continual practising of the relaxation method as described in the *Repose Recipe* and the chapter that precedes it will produce the desired results — not merely the reading of this book.

When Addiction is Feared

In those cases where there is a danger of a growing addiction to sleeping pills or other sedatives, medical opinion is usually against complete withdrawal of the drug. If you do take a pill every night in aid of instant sleep you cannot suddenly stop taking it. Psychiatrists tell us that it is no good trying to impose 'will power'; what we should do is to replace one habit by another habit . . . a more satisfactory habit.

Just because you know that sleep attained by the pill method may lead in time to addiction and also, maybe, a tolerance of the drug, requiring larger doses as the years go by, you build up an unhealthy fear of going to bed — to delay to the last possible hour the time when you must have that blessed pill. Or worse, as in the case of complete addiction, you long for your bed and the comfort of being freed from worries by the blessed pill. These are *unnatural states* and brought about by the stress and strain of the world we live in . . . the price of progress, so called. Why pay this high price personally? Who thanks you for your martyrdom?

The fears, frets and fuming blamed on the age we live in can be dispelled almost overnight by convincing yourself that in time you will be able to dispense with drugs entirely. You alone, will achieve this.

When you are practising the *Repose Recipe* your mind is taken off pills on to something else. You are replacing one habit by sowing the seeds of another. Even at your first attempts to relax you will find a glimmer of comfort and this discovery will encourage you to persist and reach for the pill less frequently . . . until one day you will realise you need it no more. Just as the gradual lessening

of alcohol or cigarettes can never lead to alco-
holism or chain-smoking so the gradual lessening of
pill-taking can never lead to addiction. But those
who require a pill only occasionally? Can they
safely put the pill bottle away, making up their
minds they are giving them up entirely? Yes. And
thank their stars the sleep course here is easy — so
much more easy than for those cases quoted above.

After consideration of hypnotism and drug
addiction, it becomes clear that the key to refreshing natural sleep is mental rather than
physical. Part of the brain never sleeps. That is the
part that awakens us when the baby cries or the
alarm clock fails to go off — that is the part
responsible for our dreams; it is what makes us
walk or talk in our sleep. You can give the
subconscious some commands to calm it before
going to sleep. Or, say the scientists, teach it to
absorb learning while one sleeps.

'Sleeping Beauty learns a language while she
sleeps,' a student friend read out to me from a
newspaper recently. 'I'd like to learn Italian — but
first tell me how I can learn to sleep!' she asked
me. The answer of course is with you here.

Now that science is starting to use sleep for its
own ends by submitting the subconscious to
instructive tape recordings (loud enough to drown
any snores, it is presumed!), the first essential is to
sleep. Personally, I consider it a crime to feed pills

to students to induce sleep whereby they might learn. Yet, however good or bad this somnolent learning may prove to be, it is certainly less fraught with danger if the sleep is a natural one, as given here, attained by reference and practice, as detailed in the two chapters that follow.

5

Comfort...Prelude to Relaxation

Clothing, Food and Bedding

I am appalled at the way some people put themselves to bed. They do not appear to consider how they dress themselves or their bed, or arrange the bedroom. Yet all we worry about in these pages are those who have to woo sleep and want to learn the natural way. For these let's stress the importance of comfort inside — out and round about.

Physical comfort bans anything that constricts anywhere — so off, men, with those pyjamas with thick collars or neckbands and elastic round the waist. And girls, off with those fabrics that are crisp, or close, clammy and unyielding to the body!

When I was finger-shopping for a trousseau nightie for an engaged girl recently, I was shocked by the number of garments that failed the 'flesh test' — harsh, prickly and everything nightwear should *not* be; and those which had reasonably soft materials were trimmed with nylon frills and prickly lace trimmings. I realise that lurex trims and nylon transparencies mean much to the modern girl and, having known none of the joys of pure silk next to her skin, she is prepared to look devastating, even if she suffers. But, by all means, let her buy this cute nightwear so long as she doesn't try to sleep in it.

In case my readers accuse me of being square-sided, I do admit that any girl should be free to look as night-sexy as she likes; twist up her hair in rubber bands, loop rings through her ear lobes, or wear a night bra or girdle. But if she must learn how to sleep, complete physical comfort becomes important, or the *Repose Recipe* will fail.

Comfort

If you must wear anything at all in bed and, personally, I think some garment is desirable for comfort, let it be loose and of silk or the nearest to silk buyable, something with an affiliation to the skin. Then, remembering that relaxation starts at the top of the head, namely the hair, see that there are no curlers or bands. The hair must be loose, free from the neck (where the small pillow can fit softly); tied with a soft ribbon loosely, if actually necessary.

Inside Comfort

But not only the outside must be right, the

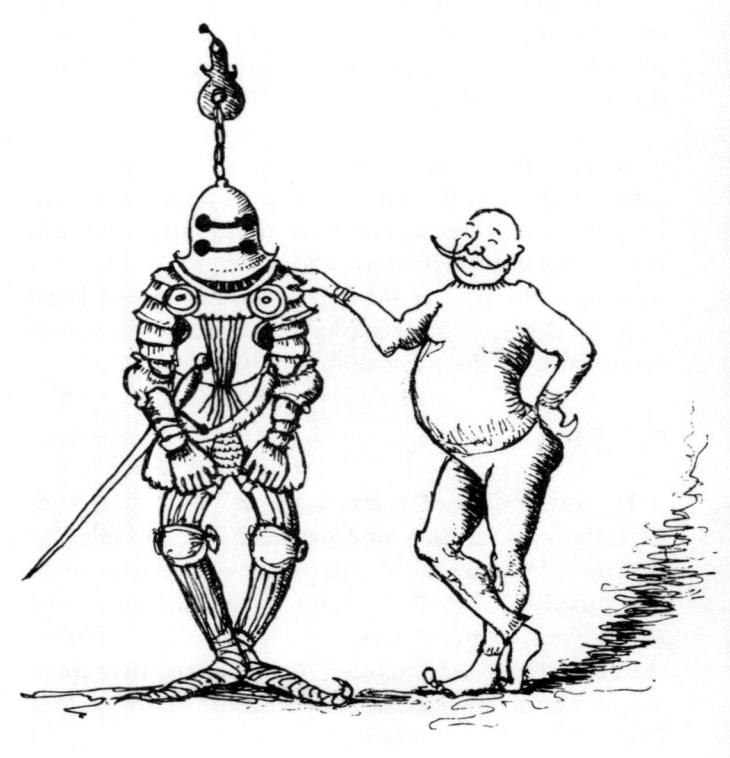

Physical comfort bans anything that constricts . . .

inside of the student must be comfortable too. Without encroaching on the medical side I may mention that normal people find it easy to 'deflate' by drawing in the stomach muscles: this can be done in the bathroom or anywhere privately. Flatulence often impedes the relaxation lesson and it is desirable that as much air should be expelled from the stomach as is possible.

For those who suffer from an empty feeling at bed-time there are the proverbial bed-time drinks based on milk. For the compulsive eater and dieter, too, (see Page 67) there must be a feeling of inner satisfaction or he will find the relaxation not as easy as he hoped. Here we refer favourably to cereal drinks obtainable from Health Food Stores; but no drink advocating any sedative or drug is suggested. Ours is the way to defeat all drugs by natural means. As for the tea and coffee, which you may decline because you feel it 'keeps you awake' — here is good news that may apply to you, one day; when I conquered the fear of sleeplessness I found I could take almost anything I wished before going to bed, tea or coffee, nightcap, or not, as my host prescribed. (You become amazingly easy to please when you master sleeplessness.)

Outside Comfort

Physically comfortable, now what is the next step?

Consider your bed. The bed itself, experts advise, should give a sleeping width not less than 36 inches or 72 inches for two; and your partner can sleep at a different temperature by providing an extra small blanket. The mattress should not squeak or sag; the bed coverings be light and warm according to the temperature but *never ever* heavy, and rather loose than too firmly tucked in. You should be free from all constriction. The pillow? The exercises demand a small, soft, sausage-shaped pillow which will take the place of your usual pillows — which can remain beside the bed in case you need them for reading in the morning; or, when you are confident and proficient in the relaxation process, you can put them under your head when almost asleep. Even after more than twenty years with this method fully mastered I find that the neck-rest pillow is essential when I now occasionally must practise the exercise. But if you have no pillow, anything soft such as a small towel, supporting the neck comfortably, allowing the head to drop over to the mattress — is possible. For example, in a train I have used silk underwear bundled into the right shape ... for nothing is more impossible for our sleep routine than train pillows; even the usual home pillows are not small or soft enough for a support to the neck.

About the Neck Cushion

Since writing this some of my readers report

that a mandarin type of neck roll helps them attain the 'head right back on the mattress' which is essential for the correct posture. Whether the neck roll is bought or home-made it is important that it fits the neck snugly and softly without any pressure. The softest foam rubber is necessary for this, cut in one piece and suitably covered in pure silk or soft cotton. The ornamental types of neck rest used for the protection of hair styles or for reading in bed are far too firm and are often made from foam scraps that form lumps: they also usually have fancy nylon covers with prickly lace trims. These are to be rejected as totally un-suitable.

The choice of the correct neck rest is mentioned here because in some cases students were per-suaded to buy the wrong type and in consequence failed to attain the very necessary comfortable posture, without which the *Repose Recipe* could not be successful.

Consider now the bedroom. Is it free from flies or mosquitos? Is it draughty or too stuffy? And is the colour scheme conducive to happiness (pastel shades of green and blue are suggested)? If you are happiest with a shielded night-light, why not have one?

Fresh air fiends, like myself, want the windows open while others prefer a warm, even temper-ature. Here the student of sleep must keep to his own way of living.

I've found that now I'm not afraid of sleeplessness, I can put up with almost anything, from the high temperature of central heating in New York to a South-Easter whipping through the ventilator of my Cape Town home. While learning, however, it is important to pander to your own idiosyncrasies for comfort preparation. But once you start on the Key Chapter, our *Repose Recipe* overleaf, there must be no deviation from the steps described.

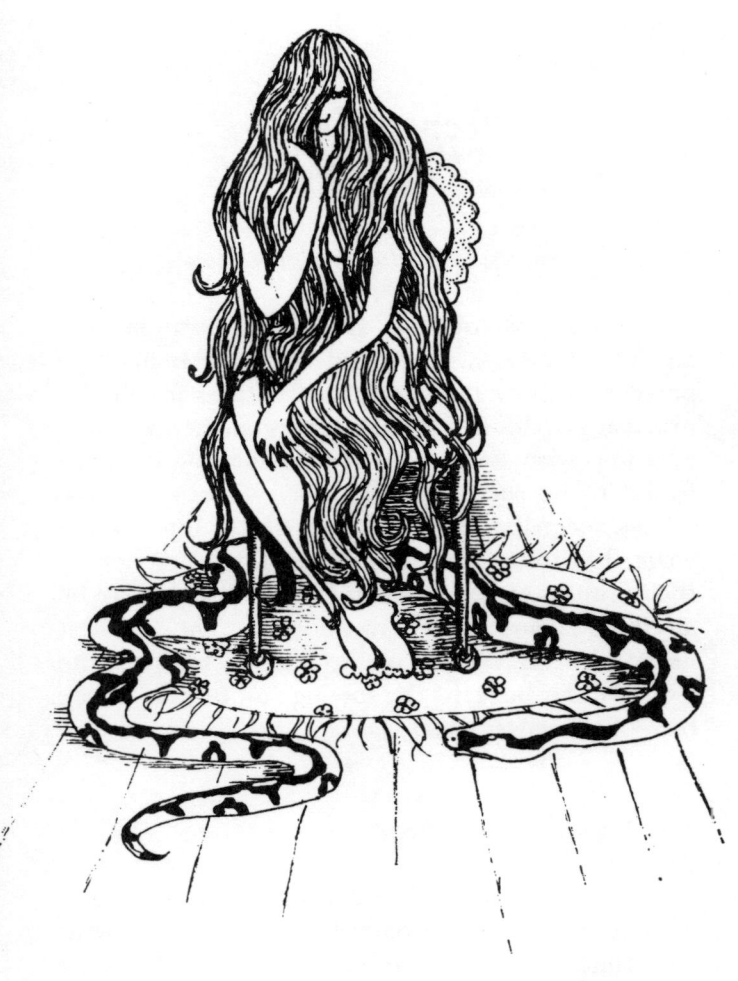

No hair bands or curlers.

6

Repose Recipe

Practise Nightly for Relaxation

The success of the following formula, the *Repose Recipe*, will depend on your being prepared to follow the simple instructions implicitly, practising without variation *every* night or whenever you wish to sleep. When the method has been found to be successful you may wish to vary the recipe according to your own taste; but, as the writer has found, it is important not to try to vary the formula at the practising stage, which may be anything from weeks to months. The smallest deviation can cause failure, loss of faith in the formula and back to the tossing and turning of the bad, old sleepless days.

You Decide to go to Bed

First make yourself comfortable for the night. This means, have your bath if you're used to one at this time, have a wam drink if you like it or anything else that makes you feel comfortable inside. Deflate flatulence by pulling the stomach muscles in and out; anoint wounds, lubricate or powder the skin. Outside, see that nightwear is comfortable; in the case of a woman, that there are no restricing hair bands or curlers or, in the case of a man, no tight pyjama collar round your neck or elastic round your waist. (Refer to Chapter *Comfort*). The bed should be comfortable too, one that doesn't creak or sag, with a firm or not too-soft mattress and adequate *light* bedding. The army recruit may sleep like a log after a hard day in the field, covered with heavy army blankets, but heavy blankets and the hard ground are not for us yet. Once sleep success has been attained, you may sleep like a soldier in the field, under any conditions almost, depending on your years!

Remember to follow the directions for comfort completely, being sure you are ready to *want* to sleep, otherwise do what you want to do before you take to your bed. Until you have mastered the method you will *not* have a notebook and pencil beside your bed to jot down office and domestic reminders. That comes when you are proficient and able to turn sleep on and off, like a tap, with complete confidence. You don't need pills or water either. All you need is the will to follow the instructions.

You Lie Down

Switch off the radio and lie flat on your back.

Don't start arguing that you can't sleep on your back — because then you will continue to argue right the way through this self-help sleep method and get nowhere. When you have succeeded in the sleep routine you will find you can always turn on your side, curl up and sleep on either side, or stomach, as you wish. So we repeat, by this method *there is no other way;* you lie flat on your back, placing one small, soft, long pillow just under the nape of the neck, and no other pillow. (See also *About the Neck Cushion*).

Now loll the head back until it touches the mattress, and start shuffling the body heavily into the bed, especially the shoulder blades; nestle the shoulders into the mattress, then relax them; you probably feel pretty awful and perhaps your legs are aching. If so — but not unless they are — place another small, soft pillow under the knees and drop back again with one pillow under the nape of the neck and one under the knees, and adjust the body as follows:

Posture

Lie limp, your head sagging back on to the mattress level, only the neck supported by the small pillow at the back of your neck. This is an unusual position, but don't rebel; you feel as if you want to open your mouth and let your jaw drop. Well, that's right — just what you *must* do. And forget about those inhibitions regarding an open mouth — the flies that might fly in, or swallowing a denture, or looking a fright. The flies and denture should have been dealt with at the 'preparing for comfort' stage and if you are self-conscious about your appearance, it may be important for you to have your own room, until you have mastered the sleep method. (Better than going to hospital with a nervous break-down anyway.)

When practising this lying-on-the-back position, the mouth opens naturally, allowing the jaw to drop and, with the dropping of the jaw, something strange happens to those stomach muscles — they appear to drop, too. Feel this to believe it! Now with jaw dropped and mouth slightly open, shut the eyes. Some find this the most difficult link in the sleep method. They even want to tie a black handkerchief over the eyes or 'see black'; but that is not our method because the handkerchief, however soft, touches the face, and 'seeing black' is using the eyes for 'seeing', which is the last thing we want them to do. Anything that restricts, hampers or makes one conscious of 'touch' is against the method. For that reason the hands are not folded across the chest as advised in some other relaxation methods, they are free of body contact.

Now look to your limbs. Slightly spread-eagle the legs and be sure that the arms do not touch the body; but the limbs need not be far flung — just

naturally lie *away* from the body. 'Go limp all
over'; the fingers will part naturally when you relax
your hand.

By now you may not feel relaxed. Instead you
may feel frustrated and helpless and some people
even think they feel faint with the head thrown
back. But in reasonably healthy people it isn't
faintness, it is merely a release of head tension and
the beginning of the good work of relaxation in
preparation for natural sleep.

The Relaxing Message

Now imagine you are sending each part of the
body to sleep, from the head to toe, while
breathing slowly and evenly — but not too deeply
if that worries you. Your eyes closed, jaw dropped,
body slightly spread-eagled on the bed, and no part
of the body touching, you can tell where the tense
spots are. Come to terms with them: Starting at
the top of the head (and your head may feel
peculiar or dizzy lolling back from the neck pillow)
concentrate on making it feel heavy, heavy,
heavier. Pass down to the eyes, making them feel
heavy, heavy, heavier. Concentrate on the eyes
until the eyelids feel almost too heavy to open
again.

The shoulders come next; although you relaxed
them into the bed when you lay down, they are

tense, and may even be aching. Shrug them and let them come to rest — again and again — heavily on the bed. Now do the same with the elbows; send them to sleep with the command — 'heavy, heavy'. Now give the same commands to the hands and the fingers. If you are not sure whether your hands are really relaxed, visualize your puppy stretched on its back with paws in the air. (Yours, of course, are relaxed slightly away from and on each side of your body on the bed; the last thing we suggest is for you to paw the air!)

By this time you'll probably be getting a little sleepy and inclined to give up this HEAVY business. But drowsily persist; and send every part of the body to sleep in turn — by relaxing into the bed; the hips, buttocks, then the calves of the legs and, lastly, the ankles and feet and toes, giving each part the special prolonged 'heavy' treatment. When you get down to the toes you may be aware of a bunion or corn throbbing. Ignore the minor pains because, in time, sleep will drug these (but make an appointment with your chiropodist on the morrow). You may also notice a tendency to pins and needles in the limbs. If so, don't worry, for this is a good sign, a sign that the body is relaxing and unaccustomed to it. In time, as you continue to practise relaxation the 'pins and needles' feeling will go.

By now you may find that the eyes are open and the jaw firmed up. So it is time to start the heavy method, step by step, all over again. But first slacken the jaw, relax the fingers, relax the mouth, let the eyes sag to a heavy close (not too tightly shut); if you sleep with eyes half open, no matter, so long as the eyes are relaxed. Yes, from top to toe, you go through the whole boring process again.

And you go on and on *every* night doing just this, instead of counting sheep or 'seeing black', or relying on a pill. It *is* boring, so boring that it works, because if you follow the instructions you have no time to think of anything else! That's why the repetition – until sleep comes – is so necessary, no other thoughts above your repetitive instructions to your body, from top to toe, can intrude. If they do, start all over again from the head, not short-cutting any of the steps given above; indeed it is better to prolong each one.

Every time the mind starts to wander you penalize yourself by starting at the top of the head again: hence the title of this book, *The Sleep Game*.

When you find yourself getting really drowsy – so drowsy that in fact you couldn't be bothered to answer the 'phone however long it rings – then you are almost asleep and can turn on to your side or whichever position you like best; pushing the neck cushion from the head, closing your mouth, even pulling another pillow to bolster your head *if* you have the energy left. And then if you awake in an hour or so? What does it matter? You go through the whole procedure again, and again.

But even when you have conquered sleeplessness you will find yourself tossing and turning sometimes, and to this day, twenty years after I did conquer sleeplessness, if particularly worried or harassed by work worries, by noise or in a high altitude I still have to practise the method in precise detail. The joy is that I now enjoy the luxury of lying awake when I want to. You will attain this freedom from fear of not sleeping too; be able to listen to the late news on the radio, come home from a party at 2 a.m., give yourself the luxury of battling with a business problem, notebook and pencil to hand; but then you will decide, 'there are only so many hours left until I must get up and I must get 6 hours sleep, at least'. Then it is you discard your pillows, reach for your 'neckrest pillow' and go through the method from top to toe again, and yet again and again if necessary. Now you'll probably find you need more than two or three top-to-toe cycles before you are drowsy and ready to turn over and sleep. You wake in an hour, maybe, and so must go through the whole process again.

In time this routine becomes auto-suggestion — a habit — and you have only to think about it in various stages to catnap or sleep on bus, plane, hospital, anywhere under almost any conditions, in fact — according to your own choice.

7

Some Special Cases

Snorers

Most people snore in some degree, at some time or other; even the most genteel, who usually claim they never snore and who would not commit themselves even to a yawn without a polite hand to the mouth. There are the intermittent mild snorers, the occasionally annoying ones and, of course, those horrific chain-gang types who qualify for all those corny jokes, such as 'they not only sleep like logs but saw them and float them down the river all through the night'. Admittedly, after having mastered the sleep problem you may discover that you have been changed from a respected insomniac into a repellent snorer. You have learnt that to acquire complete relaxation it is imperative you lie on the back with the jaw slack — which usually means the mouth is wide open; that is the exact position to acquire snoring.

According to the definition of snoring in a medical dictionary: Snoring is due to the vibration of the soft palate and 'usually occurs in mouth breathers and those who lie on the back'. To cure the snorer of assuming this position there are listed all kinds of gags and back-breaking ideas; such as tying up the lower jaw with a sling and sewing a hair brush, cotton reels, even a stone, into the lining of the patient's pyjamas! The aim being that when the snorer assumes a position on his back he will be rudely awakened and turn on to his side or stomach. But in some extreme cases — as men who have suffered snorers in cabins, aboard ship or on active service will testify — there are old campaigners at the snoring game who can be gagged, turned on to their stomachs, thrown into the air even, and yet who return to base, still snoring. When awakened they yawn and set off on another snoring campaign with gusto. Until these consult an ear, nose and throat specialist the only hope for anyone trying to sleep near them is to get as far away as possible and practise relaxation assisted by ear plugs.

Chief causes of snoring are conditions leading to blockage of the nose, and, in the case of children, enlarged tonsils and adenoids. Naturally, medical treatment consists of the removal of the causes of mouth breathing. Now how can we reconcile our sleep therapy with snoring? While I can hear the sighs of those sleep-envious bodies who desire sleep so much they don't mind how much they snore, I can hear critics of the sleep system given in this book saying 'yes, you've given a relaxation method that works maybe — but see where it leads to — snoring!' Just think of all the romances shattered

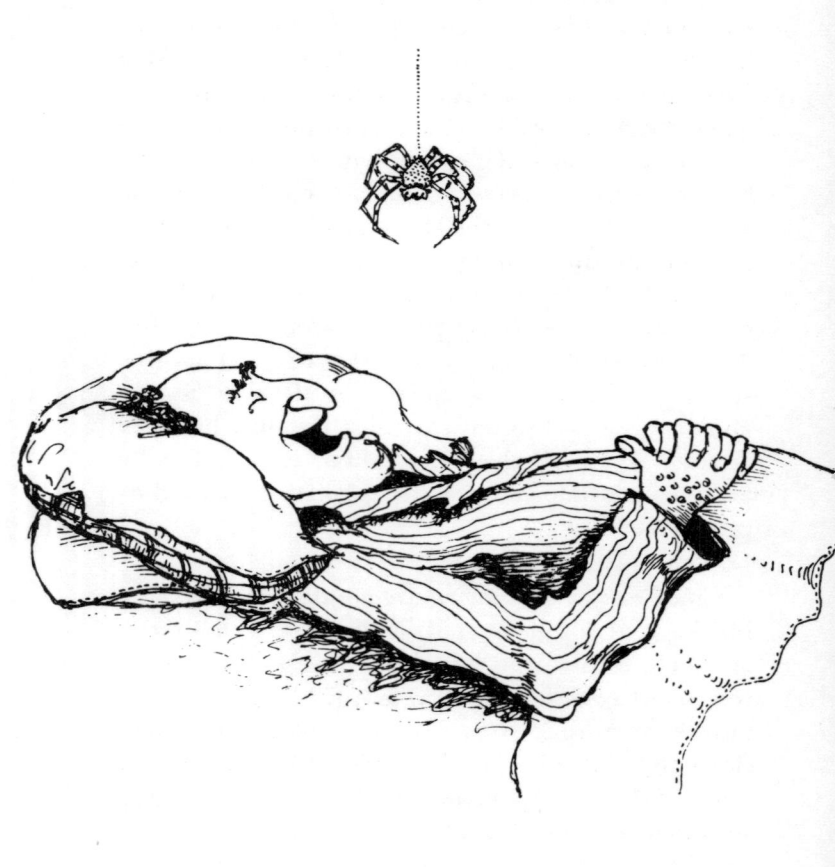

Snoring usually occurs in mouth breathers and those who lie on their back.

and marriages doomed, even from the first night of the honeymoon, where one partner discovers that the other is an incessant snorer. How often we have heard it said 'I lie awake all night, while he (or she) snores.'

My answer is that the nervous condition arising from sleeplessness is a far worse condition than that suffered by the snorer, and sleeplessness has been the cause of probably many more marriage break-downs. All the snorer needs is a separate room where he or she can snore to his or her own heart's content. What matters most to an insomniac is to learn how to sleep naturally. And as we have stressed throughout this book when completely relaxed and almost asleep you can curl up on the side or turn on to the stomach and *close the mouth*, assuming any position desired. (I must admit, however, that when I am forced to practise the relaxation exercise, because of over-tiredness or any other cause — I do wake up in the morning, more often than not, still on my back.)

In conclusion to this discussion about snoring, I go so far as to believe that it is because of the feat of lying on the back and allowing the mouth to open that many people fail to acquire the essentials of relaxation as described here and in other books. For generations, nannies and parents have discouraged this position. No wonder we are inhibited. These inhibitions must be overcome before we can hope for success.

Old Age . . . Awake!

In the latter years men and women often suffer insomnia at night because they catnap during the day. They need not feel sorry for themselves. An aunt of mine of ninety-seven complained that the nights seemed so long — until she learned to enjoy all the time she was awake, even in the middle of the night. Refer to Chapter *Old Age.*

Mothers: Your Life Line!

Mothers who must jump up and down in the night, ministering to a sick child or small baby, often set a pattern of sleeplessness for later years that increases as they approach the menopause. For their own happiness, these women should learn to turn sleep 'on and off' while they are young. The cultivation of *natural* sleep is essential. (Who dare sleep unnaturally heavily?) They will still hear the child's cry but will tend the child then drop down again, practise their relaxation and fall asleep. In time, less and less practice will be required — but the essentials given here must be regularly followed, or the art once learned will again be lost! Those mothers who have learnt relaxation for childbirth will find it easier than the others.

Weighty Problems Solved

Night eaters, according to medical men, are

often overweight people who are compelled to eat because they lie awake thinking of food. The thought becomes torture, only relieved when they go into the kitchen and open the fridge and find a snack. These unfortunate people can lose weight by practising the relaxation method for sleep described in this book. Once you are asleep you can safely afford to dream about food. The sagging jaw also achieves relaxation of the stomach muscles, and the dropping back of the head over a neck support makes one feel so helpless, one cannot be bothered to get up and hunt for food.

Catnappers

'Catnaps — do you call that sleeping?' I hear a reader ask. Of course catnappers are sleeping. Without the ability to turn sleep on and off almost as easily as you do with a water tap, you actually cannot catnap at will. (Your catnap may be just weariness or indigestion or such.) The *Repose Recipe* combined with its vital prelude *Comfort* as given in these pages ensures you get the sleep you need, not necessarily when your body needs it, but when you *decide* to indulge in sleep.

No one else, no outside influence or fee comes into the picture. Sleep is a private matter you teach yourself in private. You go to bed and say, 'I don't want to go to sleep for two hours. I really must think out this business (or domestic) problem.'

After the two hours you say sternly to yourself, 'Now is the time for me to sleep for six or eight hours because I know I really need this amount of sleep to be able to tackle the tasks of tomorrow.'

You, the Aladdin have found a lamp that can be rubbed when you will — until your dying day.

When You Cannot Read this Yourself

In those cases where for some reason the sleep student cannot read this message himself a reader should be found who can read the *Repose Recipe* (Chapter 6) slowly and clearly — even if drowsily. Warning: the one who reads it may become extremely sleepy, especially if he is reading it sympathetically.

8

Children and all Young Fry

Babies vary as to sleep needs and will usually take the amount they really require. Some babies are wakeful from the minute they are born but according to Dr. Spock, at two years the sleep habit has been formed; from then on it is advisable, if possible, that the child has a bed of his own. Personally, I consider his or her own bed is every child's birthright and the underprivileged or large families that simply cannot afford this luxury for their youngsters are to be pitied.

A wakeful child may be an exceptionally bright one or with a natural reaction to wakefulness instead of sleepfulness, or the child may be uncomfortable or unhealthy. The mother should know and the doctor will guide.

But before running to the doctor with a sleepless child why not let one's common sense decide if the child is wakeful because he is uncomfortable? After his bath, has he been made physically comfortable by a dusting powder or lubrication on what may become sore parts? If he wears a napkin, is it loose enough or has he to endure rubber pants, instead of a thin rubber sheeting *under* the soft cotton sheet on his bed, and will he be given a night change of napkin where necessary? Has he been made comfortable inside by 'burping up the wind' before he is laid down and, in the case of a small baby, moved at least once from his one side to the other during the night? On occasions when baby sitting, I've been horrified by finding a baby in a nightie too tight round the neck and with harsh turkish towelling napkins tightly pinned — trussed 'like a lamb for the slaughter', in fact.

The child when he goes to bed should feel clean and comfortable in soft, loose nightwear (not nylon) without anything prickling or constricting, no neck chains or bracelets, of course. The common sense of the mother 'feeling for her child' is the best guide here. The bed itself should have a firm mattress, the firmer the better and, for the sake of posture, without a pillow — even from the first day, and in older years compromise with one pillow only. Is the bedding light and sufficiently warm (such as cobweb wool blankets with the usual sheets)? Is the room temperature right? Airy, with the bed sheltered from draught? And, in the case of the toddler, is there sufficient light or a soft night lamp in the room to give him confidence, and the door open, so that he does not feel cut off from his parents? (Unless he is noisy when there is a threat of you closing it; this, once necessary, seldom need happen again!)

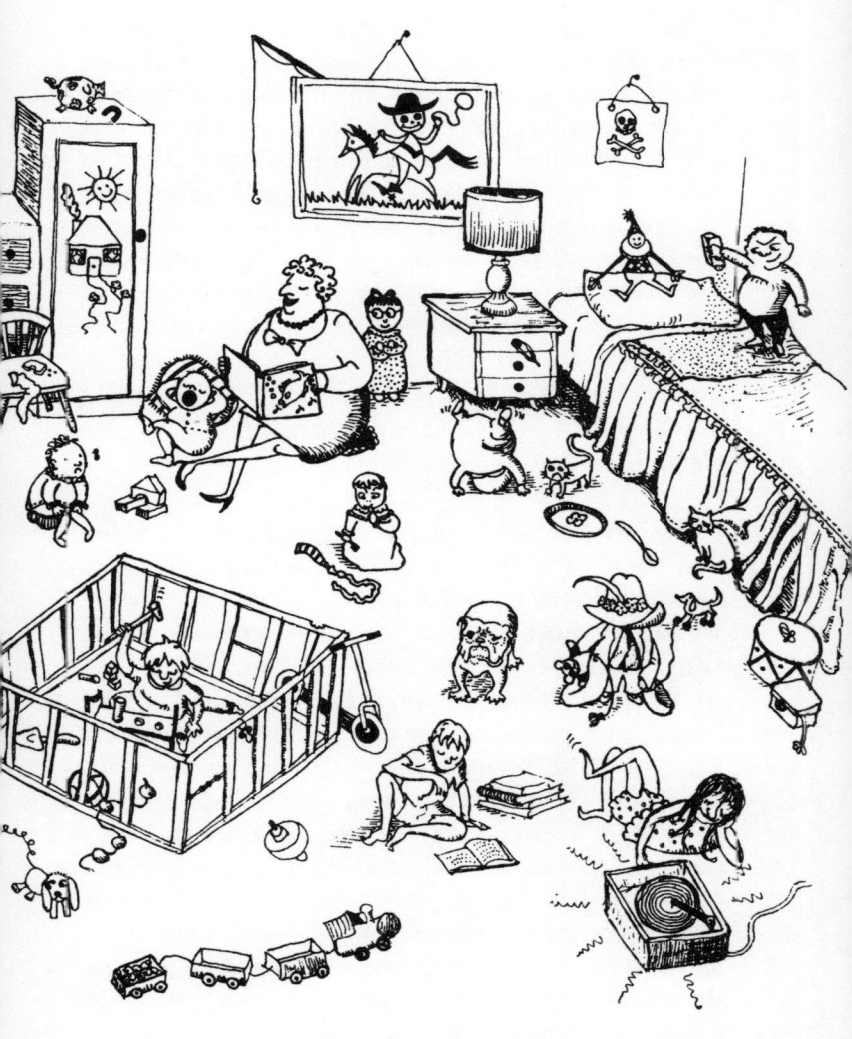

Nothing equals the bed-time story.

Naturally, among the reasonably educated at least, one expects a mother to consider such things; but in the underprivileged all the rules are broken — the children fall asleep under-nourished and often unwashed and still clothed, blissfully too tired-out to be aware of how many others are sharing their bed. Yes, only we of the affluent society must seek sleep; and yet what astonishes me is that there are so many mothers who neglect to see that their children are really comfortable when they are put to bed.

Relax with Bed-time Story

To prepare the toddler and older children for bed there is nothing equal to the bed-time story — which takes the place of the relaxation exercise we adults must practise. As an experiment, when baby-sitting in America I started out to tell a story to small children about a little fish and all its adventures, getting to the end just before bed-time, when the fish seemed sleepy and I, yawning with the fish. (There's something about fish that is soothing.) I always sit on the floor when story-telling, right down with the children; never aloof or above their heads, physically or mentally. And then it is easy to stretch yourself out on the floor and almost drop off to sleep, yawning. And just see the children (two — five) get yawny too! They will usually be already relaxed and prepared for bed before you suggest, rather half-heartedly, their beds are waiting (teeth and toilet on the way); and then — with hardly a break in the story — while they clamber into cot or bed you continue the sleepy tale: the little fish, so tired after his adventurous day, sinking right down to the bottom of the ocean and lying on the sea-bed gazing up at the sea life and the wonders of the ocean — the life in the depths as you can swot up for yourself. By this time the little fish and you, and the children, are yawning. (Have you ever tried showing a picture of someone yawning and see how they respond with their own yawns? As children I remember we cut out from a newspaper a huge picture of a yawning lion and delighted in the yawning response from our elders.) Then, still stifling a yawn, you finish off the story in a hushed voice as the fish, lying flat on his back, goes off into pleasant dreams.

Generally speaking, the children sleep right away, and, personally, I've been embarrassed at the way they tend to lie flat like a fish at the bottom of the ocean, because those prone to bed-wetting are better not on the back! If this problem is a crucial one the mother or baby-sitter can turn the child over on to side or stomach when he or she is almost asleep.

The point I wish to stress is that before one sleeps one has to be relaxed. With children, sleep comes so speedily that it almost takes one's breath away. A young child will be kicking its legs and flailing arms all over the place, then suddenly subside and, in five minutes, is asleep.

Now about this kicking. Of course they are kicking — like we older ones who 'can dance all night'. Parents know how, after an exciting or boisterous game just before bed-time, it is difficult to get the children to sleep. By all means have those boisterous games, but not just before bed-time. The last half hour or so should be the relaxation period; not a boring one by any means, but the time when little limbs rest, while they listen to an interesting story with a sleepy ending. If a child stands on his head while you're reading or telling it, no matter, he is confined to a given space and not bounding about the room. All this is part of the relaxation that we adults have to learn in the method. But the method, as described in the *Repose Recipe* in Chapter 6, is inapplicable to children; substitute the simple story relaxation as described above, which may be applied to ages from two upwards.

Sleep-Rousing Problems

The modern habit of parents taking their children out visiting with them at night, picking them up while asleep and transporting them by car from one house to another, need not be deplored. Oldsters who frown upon this practice of the 'young-marrieds' should remember that children are growing up in a very different age, a noisy age in more confined space and without the 'hush-hush' assistance of nannies. So long as the child is not talked to (except perhaps in reassuring murmurs), and not asked questions or anything that might excite his mental faculties, he will learn to doze at night through almost any smooth movements or normal noises, such as radio music or voices.

Modern life demands that we should be like these children, remain asleep by our own attitude, disregarding the noises that are with us, not only during the day, but often through the night. Remember that the country farmyard cries can distress the city folk as much as the sirens and airplanes do their country cousins. If we cultivate the relaxed attitude to sleeping we fear nothing except severe physical pain. Even this is helped by our natural sleep method, according to an arthritic woman who told me she slept well because she has always 'willed' herself to sleep. The child, father of the man, can be trained in the sleep habit that will help him throughout life.

'Now don't tell me', I can hear a parent saying, 'that the storybook method applies to children of ten, twelve and adolescents.' Yes, it does, in that everyone needs to relax before sleep. The small child who must kick in all directions at the end of the day, so keyed up is his body, is no different from the ten-year-old, so tired of battling with the family and his homework that the last thing he wants to do is lie down, much less sleep. He, like his older brothers, regards sleep as a waste of time.

The appointed bed-time hour, as laid down by the parents, must be sacrosanct. Older children must abide by that hour — nine or ten o'clock, as maybe, but they are allowed to read in bed. See that there is a suitable, easy, angle light and that they do not have to get up to switch it off, because that is in line with our relaxation method — *not* to have to move the body when it starts to relax (until relaxation for sleep is learnt, when one finds a new-found ability to get up and move about in a drowse). Let the child have a pile of books next to the bed and never forbid the light needed to read them. Nature will take its course. He'll sleep and usually turn off the light himself.

Teenagers

Teenagers? Well, I admit I've 'baby-sat' for these, too, and discovered there is nothing they long for so much as to stay up half the night. A big boast is, 'I didn't go to bed until two this morning'; and someone is sure to better that with 'three or four'. But the same relaxation rule applies. Generally speaking, teeagers will wear themselves out before wasting an hour or two in sleep. How can one appeal to them?

The only method is to promote self interest.

You can usually appeal to the girls with the old 'beauty sleep' propaganda; by suggesting they already have 'baggy eyes' and nine hours sleep is essential for good looks. And the appeal to the boys is along the lines of developing manhood: 'You could improve those muscles; nine hours sleep is necessary when you are growing to develop you properly — who wants to be a dwarf, or weakling?' And so on. You needn't expect an answer, but the message is noted and, more often than not, bears some fruit.

For the teenager the same relaxation pattern is there to follow as for the younger children. Bed at some appointed hour, say 10 o'clock, a good light and opportunity to read or listen to the radio (softly) until the body relaxes.

Nine out of ten parents will admit that their teenage children sleep long enough for good health when guided to do so, but, of course, the main aim is for them to be wide awake during school time and that means sufficient sleep at night.

Our *Repose Recipe,* Chapter 6, it will be noticed, does not apply to the very young or the very old, although the Chapter on *Comfort* — inside-out — does apply to all, as do many other observations in these pages.

As for the parents who dole out pills — even aspirin to their children on all occasions, here is a plea: don't cultivate a pill habit; show them by your example that you have learned to sleep naturally, and they can, too; even overcoming many pains, mental and physical.

9

Old Age

Sleep in the Latest Years

When I use the heading *Old Age* it is qualified by the thought that some people are old at sixty and others not quite as old at ninety-seven. I'm thinking now of an aunt, former headmistress of a London school, who came to see her sister, my mother, in Cape Town when she was ninety-two and my mother eighty-five. She came by ship, thoroughly enjoyed the voyage, using the lift from dining room to lounge where, with the windows open, she delighted in the sea breezes without the risk of breaking a leg on the sloping decks. After a holiday of six months in Cape Town she returned safely, flew from Southampton to Northern Ireland — where she passed away two years before her hundredth birthday.

My aunt confessed she would have liked to live with us in South Africa but could not bear the thought of her latter years without television, which at that time had not been introduced into South Africa. Like her brother and all the five Hazlitt sisters — one (Dr. Victoria Hazlitt) was a pioneer in psychology at London University — she was as individualistic as their father William, my grandfather, who took after a fiery ancestor, William Hazlitt, the essayist. It was a joy to talk to my aunt about anything and everything because of her keen sense of humour and common sense. Naturally, we discussed the sleep formula and how it might benefit the aged; but both came to the reluctant conclusion that the *Repose Recipe* described here might not apply to many aged people; for example, some cannot lie flat on their backs, and many must lie on the right side for the sake of the heart and digestion; supported by small cushions to buffer aching joints.

Like many old people, my aunt said she was a bad sleeper; she confessed she dreaded taking to her bed with the TV 'goodnight' and slept fitfully for only an hour or two, longing always for the dawn. In old people it seems that the built-in biological clocks that govern the 'wake and sleep' rhythm slow down like everything else; and yet trying to change a life-time pattern might do more harm than good. We talked about this over a glass of Cape wine which, in the case of my abstemious aunt, was a great adventure as she only associated wine with champagne, restricted to anniversaries and weddings. I, being fond of wines (recapturing the *vin ordinaire* days of my holidays in France), suggested if the wine agreed with her, why not take a glass before she went to bed *every* night? During her visit this became a nightly enjoyment of ours

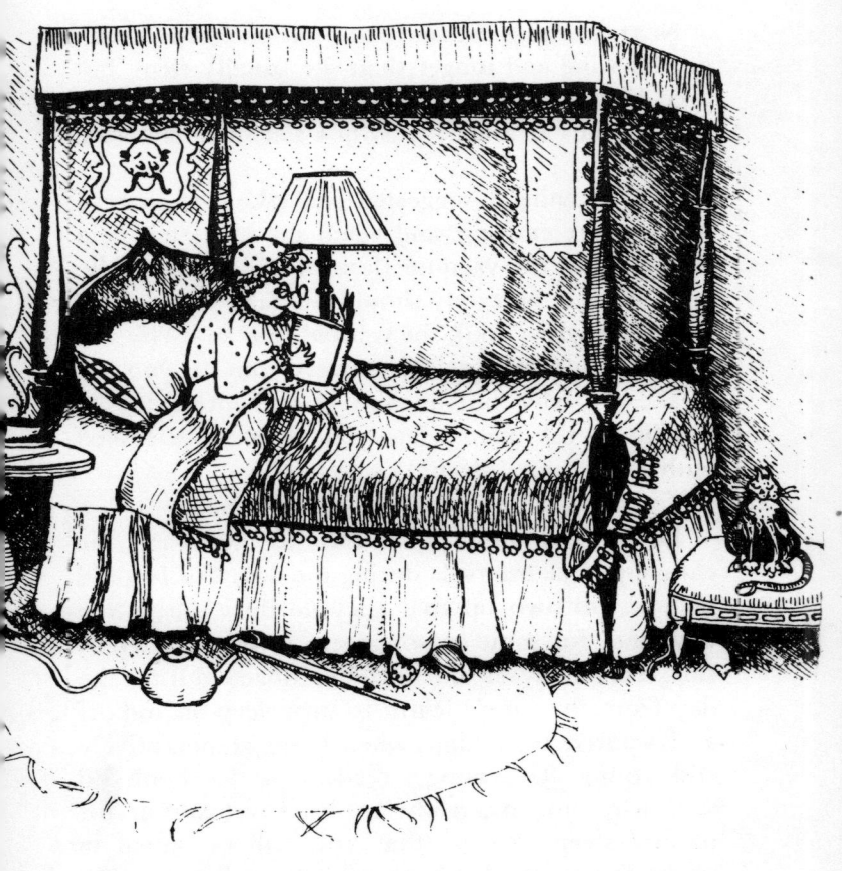

Why not spin out life a little longer?

before she retired to bed, clad in an incredible nightgown complete with an old fashioned 'money pocket'.

Next morning my aunt told me she slept better on the wine and longer than she usually slept 'but then I lay awake thinking and worrying'. 'Worrying about what?' I asked. 'Just not sleeping,' she said.

Next evening I suggested she take her glass of wine before retiring, and when she woke up, help herself from the vacuum flask of tea at the ready, near her bed. Not only should she take a cup of tea but there was a book she wanted to read. 'Why not spin out life longer, enjoy every minute you are awake . . . why not read a few chapters in the middle of the night when your eyes are refreshed with a few hours' sleep?' I suggested.

But I did not point out to her that she cat-napped at intervals during the day. For few old people will own up that they do doze during the day, and, for some reason, seem to be ashamed of·this. Personally, I am not; I've dozed during the day from the time I learnt to turn sleep on and off as I wanted to, a time when I was comparatively still young. To younger readers of this book I'd say, why not be ready to learn relaxation for natural sleep *now* so that you will be tuned in ready for your oldest years? Then when you do reach advanced years, vary the formula as suits you best and if you lie awake, learn to live a 'third' life — refreshing yourself and reading or writing or doing a jig-saw puzzle in the middle of the night. Next day you can make up with cat-naps — because if you are of advanced years you are probably not working — not at a nine till five job anyway.

Night Life

In the case of my aunt the idea worked out. When I visited her in her Irish cottage above the rocks thrashed by the wild Atlantic (about four years after her Cape Town visit), she had taken to enjoying an evening glass of wine with her kinsfolk and did not worry if she woke during the night, because then she did something she wanted to — read a few pages or polished the silver, or merely looked through her photo albums. 'I don't mind missing sleep during the night because I *do* sleep during the day,' she confessed, with a twinkle in her blue eyes. 'Since that talk we had in Cape Town, I rather enjoy my night life.' And when sitting with her in front of her TV screen in the evenings, I noted how she loved 'living with the news'; every minute of the Queen's visit to Germany, the Grand National, the Boat Race; then, when she became bored, she dozed. Why not? When you have cast out the fear of not sleeping, you of any age, can doze as you will, and in the case of old age, without apology.

In Conclusion

Even now, more than twenty years after acquiring the ability to sleep when and as I wish, there are many nights I have to practise the method, step by step, as described in the *Repose Recipe*; the occasions being when I am particularly distressed by bad news, over-tired, or pressured by problems or too much work, or visiting at a high altitude. Yet with the ability which comes with practice — sleep is at hand always to be turned off and on just when needed.

If you want to think about pressing problems at the office, well, you can give yourself this 'luxury' of one or two hours as you may wish and then, looking at the clock, decide, *'Now* I must sleep'. How? By practising the simple *Repose Recipe*, Chapter 6, which will stand by you until your dying day — made easier because of it — and *without* that sleeping pill.

One in ten persons in Britain takes a sleeping pill every night. Not only middle-aged and old people, young people too.

There was a girl of twelve who, because she was unhappy at home, took some of her mother's sleeping pills when she went to bed. She increased the number until she was taking a score and more pills every night, and a few years later was put into custody as a hard drug addict (LSD), her life hanging by a thread.

There are many cases today where drug addiction started with a sleeping pill — far, far more than when I started writing this book. For that reason I implore parents and teachers to study the natural sleep method described in detail here. Learn to relax and sleep naturally yourselves. The strains and stresses peculiarly applicable to the world of today demand that we learn to sleep. The dangers of drug addiction demand that we learn to give up tranquillizers and sleeping pills. While we ourselves use potentially dangerous artificial means to get us through life we can hardly expect our children and pupils to forego similar 'crutches'. It is these small crutches, 'pill popping' for every pain or fear, that lead to a craving for stronger and harder stuff. A way of life that is threatening our generation may kill off the next more effectively than atomic fall-out!

I know couples who think nothing of giving their babies tranquillizers nightly for those special occasions such as Christenings 'to be sure he doesn't cry'. (*They* are the ones who should be crying!) There is the case of a mother who buys packets of children's aspirin for her seven-year-old and tells him to keep them in his pocket and take one whenever he feels toothache or headache coming on. People I know who are against alcohol take sleeping pills regularly and give them to their children. Both are drugs.

Why do they do it?

The answer is clear; they don't believe they themselves can live without these crutches and that is why they prove so inadequate when dealing with drug addiction later on in the case of their own youngsters.

Yet there is a happy way to woo sleep that costs nothing beyond the effort of nightly practice, observing the rules given in these pages.

Over twenty-five years ago if anyone had told me I'd be able to learn how to turn sleep on and off like a water tap, I would have scoffed 'all that mumbo jumbo, self-hypnosis stuff, not for me'. That was before the tragedy that compelled me to find a natural means of sleeping . . . before the mystery that consumed my entire life, the disappearance of my husband in naval uniform without trace when on leave in 1945. (The mystery remains unsolved to this day.) My need for some sleep was so great, my sanity and job and children's education so seriously threatened, that I had to persevere in finding a way. I was scared of taking pills because all my senses had to be alert to help the police in their search and deal with all the friends, mediums, 'nuts' and others who offer help at such tragic times.

Miraculously it seemed, some simple rules found in a 'condensed book' that I applied did seem to help me attain some form of relaxation. As the weeks and months went by I decided I might as well go on practising them, adapting them to my own requirements and introducing what I considered some essential rules for comfort as a prelude to practising the *Repose Recipe*.

Since then I have proved without doubt that the natural sleep method I evolved for myself throughout the years is the happiest of all escapes from the torture of insomnia.

But could others be helped to the same degree? Each of us has his own private hell and so many are subject to actual pain, mental and physical, always more acute at night.

My demonstrations to University students reassured me that others could benefit in a similar way. Then the letters of success started to arrive. These were about fifteen per cent of all the letters I received, most of which were from people trying out the method and hoping for success. Three letters selected from scores of those received follow. They are from writers poles apart in their

problems, yet suffering from that common complaint — a need for sleep. These people are working
at it and succeeding. To each of them I had
stressed the importance of reading the book three
times, then practising the *Repose Recipe*, nightly,
step by step; particularly observing the necessity
for relaxing the jaw (even if the mouth opens); and
that all-important rule, when the mind wanders
from the exercise, of penalizing oneself by starting
at the top of the head all over again, again and
again.

Dear Mrs. Heard,

Thank you for your letter of the 2nd instant and your book the 'sleep game', for which I enclose Postal Orders value R1.50.

A local man, the late Mr. Laz Barnett, who was a very good hypnotist also told me my trouble was that I couldn't relax and told me to try the relaxing game only starting from the feet up but he didn't say anything about the posture you describe. I did try it but it wasn't always successful.

Anyway I haven't slept so quickly or so well for years as I have done this week since trying your method. Even though owing to severe Arthritis in the upper part of my spine and neck I can't drop my head back over a pillow. I make myself comfortable on my soft pillow and follow the rest of your instructions. It is really wonderful to have 8 and even 9 hours sleep a night after being used to only between 3 and at the most 6 hours.

Once again many thanks.

Yours sincerely,

(Mrs.) G.S.

Dear Mrs. Heard,

I thank you most sincerely for your letter and book The Sleep Game.

I would like to tell you that this book has helped a great deal already. At first it was hard going, and I was waking up all night, but went back to sleep again shortly after when I practised the instructions. I was taking two sleeping tablets each night, I now am taking one and gradually I am trying to do without the other, which I know will come in time.

I am enclosing herewith a postal order to the value of R1.50 for your book.

Strangely enough I was never a person who could sleep on my back, I always had the most terrible nightmares when I did. Now I find that I do fall asleep much quicker when I lie on my back and I do not get these nightmares anymore. I suppose it must have just been imagination.

Thanking you again. I will write later on and let you know how I am getting on.

Yours faithfully,

(Mrs.) P. de B.

Dear Mrs. Heard,

What a joy it is after nearly sixty years of a sleep starved life to the learning to sleep.

My record is 7¼ hours, followed the next night with 3, 2, 1 and 3, 2 the third night. There are many nights when I just can't fall asleep. One night I carried out the recipe for nearly 4½ hours and gave up. Soon after I was asleep! On another night it must have been about six a.m. before I fell asleep, but the sleep was very deep as I did not hear the alarm go off (the first time in my life for sure) and was late for work and didn't CARE!

Another aspect which gives me great thankfulness now is that I sometimes have a desire to go to bed at 10 p.m. Previously I did not care when I went to bed, 12 midnight, 1 or 2 a.m., lying awake was an agony of hopelessness. When I was a young man I would run miles and miles and walked great distances to try and induce sleep without success. I was at P.E. then and could do the Marine Drive, 26 miles, walking, in about 5 hours. This kept me physically fit and saved my sanity. During the cold months I still go for a run at night as I find this shakes off any tensions of the day.

I think I mentioned before that I had a collection of books on sleep, insomnia etc. Some are very good and I can appreciate their message much better now because of your little book which, in its way, is a masterpiece. I am so glad you decided to write the book and specially the way you did, I love the humorous bits and the drawings. I am not just saying this but the little book is the most beneficial investment I have ever made. It has paid rich dividends.

With kindest regards.

Very sincerely,

(Mr.) B.B.